THE NEW SELF HELP SERIES

PROSTATE TROUBLES

A comprehensive self help programme of diet,
exercise and natural therapies which will
enable any man to prevent the onset of
prostate troubles, or to bring relief and hope
to those already suffering.

THE NEW SELF HELP SERIES

PROSTATE TROUBLES

A DRUG-FREE PROGRAMME
TO HELP ALLEVIATE
PROSTATE PROBLEMS

LEON CHAITOW
ND DO

Thorsons
An Imprint of HarperCollinsPublishers

Thorsons
An Imprint of HarperCollins*Publishers*
77–85 Fulham Palace Road,
Hammersmith, London W6 8JB

Published by Thorsons 1988
9   10

© Thorsons Publishing Group Limited 1988

Leon Chaitow asserts the moral right to
be identified as the author of this work

A catalogue record for this book
is available from the British Library

ISBN 0 7225 1561 8

Printed in Great Britain by
HarperCollinsManufacturing Glasgow

Contents

1.

The Prostate — Its Structure and Function

For many men the problems which are common with the prostate gland present serious health complications, affecting not only their lives but often the lives of their families too. Medical research has shown that one man in two will develop prostatic hypertrophy (enlargement of the prostate gland) between the ages of 40 and 60. The optimistic view of this rather dismal statistic is that one man in two will *avoid* prostate problems. This implies that prostate problems are not inevitable, not simply a 'part of growing older'. It would also suggest that it might be possible to isolate the reasons for the difference between those men who do and those who do not develop an enlarged prostate, with all its associated difficulties.

We will go on to examine the various types of prostate problems and their concomitant symptoms later in the book, but first it might be helpful to study the structure and function of this important but somewhat mysterious gland.

In the adult man a healthy prostate is about the size and shape of a walnut. It is partly muscular and partly glandular in construction, and is located at the base of the bladder, at the point where the urethra — the tube which drains urine from the bladder — joins. Its broad upper surface lies just behind the pubic bone, and it narrows in shape to an apex through which the urethra passes along with the ejaculatory ducts. Its major function is to produce a fluid which acts as a carrier for sperm; without this fluid a man would be sterile.

The position of the prostate means that should it become enlarged the consequences can be twofold: first any swelling squeezes the urethra, causing difficulty in passing urine; second such enlargement may also restrict the passage of spermatic fluid resulting in problems with fertility. Although this in itself need not result in sexual dysfunction, the bladder problems which are often associated with an enlarged prostate can lead to impotence.

At birth the prostate is largely undeveloped, but by puberty it will have almost doubled in size as the secondary sexual characteristics, such as body and facial hair, and deepening of the voice, occur. During the years up until about the age of 30, there is a continuing development of the glandular aspect of the prostate, after which time one of two things happen: either a gradual atrophy occurs and the gland shrinks in size; or, the opposite may take place, and it

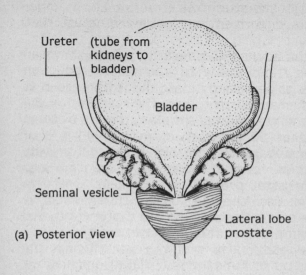

Ureter (tube from kidneys to bladder)

Bladder

Seminal vesicle

Lateral lobe prostate

(a) Posterior view

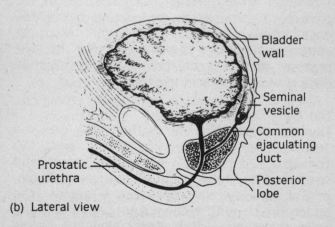

Bladder wall

Seminal vesicle

Common ejaculating duct

Posterior lobe

Prostatic urethra

(b) Lateral view

Fig 1   The prostate gland

gradually increases in size.

It would seem entirely logical and natural that the gland, which is a major component of sexual reproduction, should begin to reduce slowly in size as the primary function of reproduction passes its peak, and indeed this is the case in at least half of all men. It is the reasons for the failure of this normal shrinking to take place, in the other 50 per cent of males, which is of paramount importance. For these will provide the clues to the successful prevention and treatment of prostate enlargement. One area that has been shown to be particularly effective in the prevention of prostate dysfunction, and in the improvement of prostate problems where they already exist is diet — in particular the correction of fundamental dietary imbalances, and this aspect will be discussed in detail in the following chapters.

In order to understand fully the role of the prostate, it is necessary to examine briefly the male genital system. This will help our understanding of the vulnerability of the prostate and the reasons for its dysfunction having such far-reaching effects.

The Male Genital System
This comprises the testes (testicles); the vas deferens; the seminal vesicles and the ejaculatory ducts as well as the penis and scrotum. The male germ cell, the spermatazoa, is produced by the reproductive glands, the testes, which hang in the scrotal bag outside the abdominal cavity. This means that the testes are maintained at a temperature which is a

degree or two below that of the body as a whole and this is important for sperm production.

The spermatazoa are formed in that part of the testis known as the body. From here they pass into the epididymis, which in turn leads to a muscular sperm duct or the vas deferens. The two ducts (one from each testis) pass through the spermatic cord into the inguinal canal and on into the abdominal cavity. Here the ducts leave the spermatic cord to pass into the pelvis, behind the bladder and into the prostate, where they link with the seminal vesicles (which produce some of the transport fluid for the sperm) to form the ejaculatory duct.

The ejaculatory ducts run through the posterior part of the prostate gland, and finally open into the prostatic urethra.

The secretion produced by the prostate is squeezed into the urethra just prior to ejaculation; here it is mixed with the suspension of spermatazoa and the fluid produced by the seminal vesicles. The final mixture is called seminal fluid and this is what is ejaculated during sexual intercourse.

A healthy prostate allows free micturition (passing of urine) as well as sexual function. To present a programme which maintains this highly desirable state of affairs, and promotes full recovery if problems are already manifest, is the main aim of this book.

Recent research has shown that prostate problems are increasing dramatically. At the turn of the century they were rare and yet now prostate problems are a common complaint in the elderly citizens of the USA and Europe. This would imply a direct link between the way of life, and in particular the diet, of twentieth-century man and dysfunction of the prostate and that the solution must therefore lie in a radical alteration of that way of life and diet. It is not by chance that the only animals to suffer in any significant numbers from prostate problems are dogs. The unnatural dietary and general conditions of life of many dogs, reflecting that of their masters, makes this understandable, since these are the very factors which are largely responsible for the condition in man as well.

When the prostate is abnormally enlarged, and causing problems such as those which are discussed in the following chapter, surgery is often the medical answer. Such an approach, however, is in no sense of the word a cure. It simply excises the offending gland, sometimes with less than satisfactory results. The tragedy of this approach has been that it has largely blinded medical science to the possibility of an effective *preventive* approach. Since it is possible to simply remove the gland, why bother to stop it from enlarging in the first place?

This is a very similar story to that associated with tonsils. For many years these were removed surgically almost as soon as they became a problem. Nowadays of course the folly of such an approach has been driven home by the indisputable evidence that such operations lead to a greatly decreased resistance to infection. Tonsils are only removed now as a last resort.

Yet tonsils were always amenable to a dietary

approach which detoxified the body and so reduced the work load placed on these filtration organs. In a similar manner the prostate is amenable to a nutritional approach, which provides it with essential nutrients. It is a deficiency in such essential nutrients that is the major precursor of prostate enlargement. This means that there are effective measures that any individual can take to ensure a great deal of protection from the danger of an enlarged prostate. There are also effective treatments which can be used to reduce the troublesome symptoms of a prostate if it has already enlarged, without resorting to surgery. Once we have established the types of problem to which the prostate is prone we will move on to an investigation of these methods.

2.

Possible Problems of the Prostate

There are two major forms of prostate problem which experience has shown are responsive to self-help measures: first, prostatitis, an inflammation and usually infection of the prostate gland; and second, hypertrophy of the prostate, where the gland enlarges, resulting in a variety of unpleasant symptoms which we will discuss below. The enlargement of the prostate is also known, more accurately, as benign prostatic hypertrophy (BPH) and this is the term which we will use henceforth.

There is of course a third possible disease of the prostate, cancer of that organ, but this is not within the scope of a self-help book. Cancer of the prostate is the major form of cancer affecting the reproductive system of males. Preventive measures (these are outlined in later chapters,) will almost certainly stop the gland degenerating from simple enlargement to a state of malignancy. Such a progression is by no means inevitable, although malignancy seldom occurs unless the gland has displayed enlargement (BPH) previously.

Acute Prostatitis

In some cases acute prostatis is the result of a sexually transmitted agent, such as venereal disease. This is, however, not the major cause of prostatitis which usually derives from an infection in some other part of the body. The presenting symptoms are usually a combination of fever (102°F 38.9°C) and flu-like aches, together with shivering. This is accompanied by aching in the back and between the legs, with major discomfort felt on sitting. There will also be a great deal of discomfort or even pain on passing water and during bowel movements.

Medical treatment usually involves bedrest and a course of antibiotics for about 10 days with copious amounts of liquid, followed by a further week or so of rest. During the entire course of treatment no alcohol or sexual activity are allowed. Recurrence of the problem is common if the rules of rest and diet are not followed.

There is also a chronic form of prostatitis, triggered usually by a persistent infection of some part of the body such as the teeth or the tonsils. This produces recurring attacks of slight fever, sexual difficulties and an ache in the low back as well as between the legs and in the back passage. Medical treatment usually involves a course of sulpha drugs and massage of the prostate.

There is a close relationship between bladder infection and prostatitis as well as urethritis, an inflammation of the urethra. It is difficult to distinguish these conditions, especially as they often coexist, despite the fact that prostatic fluid contains an antibacterial factor which inhibits infection. (This probably accounts for the fact that men have less urinary infection than women.)

Prostatitis may occur at any age, although it is commoner in later years as the chances of BPH increases. Thus it can be seen that one of the precursors of an inflamed prostate is an enlarged one, although there are other possible causes. In older men the presenting symptoms of prostatitis may not involve any fever, but may simply be a degree of urgency in wanting to pass water, with an accompanying hesitancy or difficulty in controlling the flow. In such cases bacteria are usually found to be present on culture of the urine. Other men may present with symptoms such as frequency of urination, difficulty in urination, foul smelling urine, as well as cramp-like sensations in the loins, etc. In many cases the only symptoms of an inflamed prostate are vague sensations of discomfort in the lower back and mild difficulty on urination.

There are a number of self-help methods which have proved extremely effective in the treatment of prostatitis, including detoxification diets, and supplements of specific nutrients such as vitamin C (in very high doses) and zinc. These self-help methods are dealt with fully in the following chapters.

Benign Prostatic Hypertrophy (BPH)

Prostate conditions are a major health problem throughout the developed countries. Yet such conditions are hardly known in the underdeveloped world. This can only lead to the conclusion that the causes of such conditions lie in the diet or lifestyle of industrialized man.

The first indication of an increase in the size of the prostate is usually a painless increase in the frequency of passing water. A man will suddenly find that he has to urinate, often at about 2 or 3 a.m. at night. Eventually the need to pass water will become more urgent and more frequent, affecting both day and night, until other symptoms are noted, such as a difficulty in commencing urination. Any attempt at straining is useless and can have a further detrimental effect by increasing the pressure in the lower abdomen, so reducing the flow even more. Once urination has commenced, control of the noticeably weaker urine stream may become difficult, ending in a dribble which may take some time to stop. There may or may not be sexual difficulties associated with prostate hypertrophy, although usually such difficulties are connected with associated infection, or other accompanying conditions.

The enlarged prostate may be pressing on the urethra, restricting the flow of urine and making control of urination difficult. If the enlargement is marked it may result in the prostate blocking the opening of the bladder into the urethra, thus obstructing the flow of urine completely. The more effort exerted, the more blocked the passage of urine becomes. It is possible for the strength of the peak stream of urine to be tested medically, or you can test it yourself with the help of some inexpensive equipment obtainable from most pharmacists.

Urine Flow Rate Test

- If the need to urinate increases in frequency to more than five times in 24 hours;
- If you experience sudden, abrupt stopping of the urine flow during urination;
- If there is an obvious weakening of the force of the flow of urine;
- If the stream of urine becomes noticeably thinner;
- Or if you feel any pain, or pass any blood, during urination, then it might well be wise to seek medical advice and it is imperative to embark on self-help measures if deterioration is to be avoided and improvement achieved. Apart from any other consideration a reduced flow of urine may result in a small amount of urine being left in the bladder, giving rise to infection which could even result in damage to the kidneys. Thus it is very important that problems concerned with urination are resolved.

Testing the flow rate of urine for yourself also provides a valuable guide to progress as treatment or self-treatment continues.

Normally flow rate is measured in millilitres per second (ml/sec) (28 millilitres constitute 1 ounce). The rate is measured also in volume, the amount of urine passed at any time. Older men usually have a slower flow rate if the prostate is enlarged, but this may also be due to other factors, such as weakened or sagging musculature. The average flow rate is between 10 and 32 ml/sec.

You can purchase a urine flow meter from a pharmacist (it may need to be ordered). This consists of a cup with a foam lining to prevent any splattering of the urine. Below the cup is a scale on which is measured the rate of flow, and beneath that is a collection bag into which the urine flows. The instructions accompanying the meter should be followed precisely, especially not to shake or alter the upright position of the unit. It is usually desirable for a pint or two of water to be consumed some four hours prior to the test, since unless a good quantity of urine is passed the test will not be accurate. No straining should be employed during the test.

Various problems will result in a reduced urine flow rate, including narrowing of the urethra from an old infection; stones in the kidneys; bladder or other tumours, or the consequences of neurological damage to the area. However the most likely cause in middle-aged men is BPH.

Other Symptoms and their Implications
As well as the alteration to the urine flow, there may well be the development of associated symptoms, such as pain in the lower abdomen, or between the legs, in the back or, as in sciatica, in the legs only. The strength of the symptoms varies from person to person; in some they may be slight, in others very marked. If such associated symptoms arise over a period of weeks, rather than months, then medical

advice should be sought as the problem may involve more than simple enlargement of the prostate (BPH), which is usually pain- and symptom-free, apart from the urinary difficulties already discussed.

Note: It should be clear that the advice given in this book relating to BPH is not intended to be used in cases of prostate cancer. BPH stands for *benign prostate hypertrophy,* the word benign indicates that the enlargement (hypertrophy) of the gland is not malignant. Check your symptoms against the summary below and answer the following questionnaire. If in any doubt, consult your doctor.

Summary of Symptoms of BPH

- Progressive urinary frequency.
- Urgency, especially at night.
- Hesitancy and lack of control of passage of urine.
- Difficulty in cessation of passage of urine (dribbling).
- Reduced force of urine stream.
- Enlarged non-tender, non-lumpy prostate.
- Possible presence of blood in the urine if obstruction is prolonged.
- Possible associated infection of bladder due to stagnant urine.

Prostate Self-assessment Questionnaire

Answer the following questions with a *yes,* meaning this is almost always so; or a *sometimes* meaning that this is the case once a week or more, but not constantly; or *rarely,* if less than weekly. Do not answer if *no.*

Score 3 points for a *yes* answer, 2 points for a *sometimes* answer and 1 point for a *rarely* answer.

Q1. Do you have difficulty in urinating, whether it's starting the flow or stopping it (i.e. a dribble continuing for some time) or notice a burning sensation when passing urine?
   yes/sometimes/rarely

Q2. Do you have to get up at night to pass water?
   yes/sometimes/rarely

Q3. If you answered yes to either Q1 or Q2, do you feel any discomfort in the lower back, loins or back of the legs when urinating?
   yes/sometimes/rarely

Q4. Have you noticed a diminishing, or loss of, sexual drive?
   yes/sometimes/rarely

Q5. Have you been told by your doctor that you have a prostate enlargement?
   yes/no

Scoring
0 to 2 indicates no real problem.
3 to 5 indicates a problem and that the advice in this book should be heeded. A checkup or examination would also be recommended, if improvement is not noted within a month or so of introducing the nutritional (zinc supplementation, etc) programme as outlined, later in the book. A score which is above 5 indicates prostate dysfunction and calls for an immediate medical examination. Start the self-help programme straight away in conjunction with your medical advice.

This self-assessment is not meant to take the place of responsible advice from a health-care practitioner, but is a guide to the possible current state of prostate enlargement. It may be repeated from time to time (not less than monthly intervals) in order to aid in assessment of progress as the self-help programme is undertaken.

We will next consider a method of examination of the prostate by direct finger contact. This is *not a self-administered* examination, but requires a co-operative and gentle friend or family member. It is not essential but is useful, both for keeping a check on progress during self-treatment, and as an actual form of treatment by prostate massage.

3.

Examination and Massage of the Prostate

It is standard practice for a doctor to check the health of the prostate gland by feeling its contours and texture during a medical examination. This is known as palpation. There is nothing to prevent such an examination being done by a friend or member of the family, in order to provide guidance as to the degree of hardness, enlargement and subsequent improvement, in the gland. Examination and/or massage of the prostate involves the gentle insertion of a gloved finger into the rectum, in a precise manner, and this obviously calls for a degree of mutual trust and respect.

The Normal Prostate
The normal gland is about the size of a walnut with two lobes (as in a shelled walnut) and a central groove. It should therefore feel about 1 to $1\frac{1}{2}$ inches in length, with a shallow groove in

the midline. The correct consistency has been described as the texture you feel if you make a tight fist, and then with the other hand feel the muscular tissue which lies between the base of the thumb and the base of the index finger (see fig 2). This is a muscular but not rock hard texture; neither is it soft and mushy.

Examining the Prostate Manually

It is best if the person to be examined empties his bladder and bowels before the examination starts (although it is still likely that an urge to pass urine will be felt during the examination). Then he should kneel on the floor before a low bed and rest his chest and abdomen on the bed so that he is quite comfortable and relaxed.

An alternative position is for the person being examined to lie on the bed, facing the edge, with his knees tucked up to his chest. The examiner then stands in front of the person and, by leaning over his pelvic area, can carry out the examination.

The examiner should wear surgical gloves (most chemists sell these) and lubricate the index finger — the examining one — with a sterile gel such as Vaseline or K-Y. Never use anything to lubricate which is medicated or perfumed. Check that the nail of the examining finger is well trimmed to avoid the possibility of scratching or causing unnecessary discomfort.

The examiner should then press the examining finger gently against the person's anus. At first no effort should be made to penetrate the rectum. As the external muscles relax, he should insert the finger, gently but

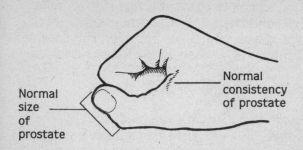

Fig 2   Guide to checking size and consistency of
the prostate gland

firmly, to its limit. If any resistance is felt, no
force should be used, but wait for the muscles
to relax. Once the examiner has penetrated the
rectum, he should press downwards lightly with
the pad of the finger tip and it should be
possible to feel a walnut-sized mass; this is the
prostate gland.

If the length of the gland does not seem
excessive, no more than $1\frac{1}{2}$ inches say, then it is
probably not enlarged or only very slightly so. In
some cases it can reach the size of an orange. It
should feel smooth and firm to the examining
finger, not soft and mushy, or hard and nodular.
The examiner should be able to detect the
midline groove. If the prostate feels lumpy
(nodular) and very hard, then medical advice
should be sought.

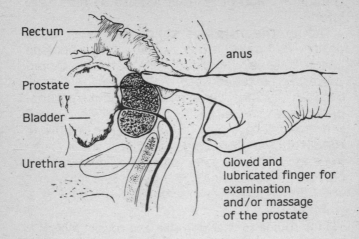

Rectum

anus

Prostate

Bladder

Urethra

Gloved and
lubricated finger for
examination
and/or massage
of the prostate

Fig 3　Manual examination of the prostate

Massaging the Prostate

While the subject is in the examination position,
it is possible to massage the gland lightly, by
gently but firmly stroking the gland, as though
it were being milked of its contents. The
examiner should use a series of slow, steady
strokes, working from the furthest end of the
gland towards the rectum (i.e. the finger should
be drawn towards the examiner). In doing this
massage the lobes of the gland, as well as the
groove between them, and also the area where
the lobes attach to surrounding tissue, should
all receive several firm, slow-moving pressure
strokes from the pad of the palpating finger.
This should take no more than a minute. Such
massaging can greatly assist in normalizing a
congested gland, especially when combined with

the dietary and other methods to be discussed later.

During the massage there may well be a desire to pass urine which may become uncontrollable. Suitable precautions should therefore be taken before the massage starts, such as placing disposable absorbent material underneath the subject.

If the prostate palpates as nodular or lumpy, then it should not be massaged. Nor should it be massaged if it is very soft and slushy. Only perform the massage if the gland feels firm and not lumpy, but enlarged beyond the size of a walnut.

The massage can be done once or twice a week during the treatment phase, and examination can be carried out once a fortnight or so to assess the improvement which will usually be noted as the gland slowly returns to a normal size.

Subsequent to massage of the prostate there may be noted a distinct improvement in the control of passing of urine. This may be only temporary at first, but if the dietary and other methods outlined in the next chapter are also being used, this should steadily become permanent.

4.

The Role of Nutrients in the Health of the Prostate

In this chapter we will take a general look at some of the nutrients which are vital in the safe self-help treatment of (and, of course, in the prevention of) prostate problems. Later in the book we examine in detail the evidence for their value, as well as providing information as to sources and amounts required. But for now, we present an outline of the sorts of nutrients and the ways in which these are known to affect underlying biochemical changes.

It is sometimes believed that as there are so many different nutrients which are useful in dealing with the prostate any one of these is adequate to the task of normalizing the gland. However, the fact is that there are a number of vital nutrients, which should be used together in the diet, taken either in food, the ideal way, or as supplements, the practical manner of ensuring an adequate intake.

The prostate gland is a very complex organ and its function involves a variety of factors interacting in a carefully balanced system. The changes which are involved in BPH represent an imbalance in this network which is related to the presence of, and interaction between, male hormones such as testosterone, and other hormones and substances such as prolactin, oestradiol, etc.

The first named of these, testosterone, decreases in its presence in the body from the age of about 40, whereas the others increase at this time. The ultimate effect of these changes in older men is often to increase the presence in the prostate of a derivative of testosterone called dihydrotestosterone (DHT). Normally DHT is excreted from the gland in sufficient quantities to prevent enlargement occurring and to maintain the prostate at its normal size. However if there should be an imbalance between the hormones, and this is common in later life, DHT is not adequately excreted, causing the prostate to swell. When an enlarged prostate is examined it is possible to detect three or four times the normal levels of DHT.

Nutrients such as the mineral zinc as well as a high protein intake have been shown to reduce the levels of, or the activity of, an enzyme which aids in the conversion of testosterone to DHT. This enzyme is known as 5-alpha reductase, and its activity increases (making prostate enlargement more likely) when the diet is high in carbohydrates and low in protein. Its activity is reduced (thus decreasing the likelihood of prostate enlargement) when the diet is high in protein and low in carbohydrate. Similarly, when zinc levels are high the activity of 5-alpha reductase is lowered, thus reducing the chance of prostate enlargement occurring. Unfortunately zinc levels in modern man are seldom adequate, and so with this deficiency comes an increase in 5-alpha reductase levels, leading to high levels of the testosterone derivative DHT, and so an enlargement of the prostate. (We will be looking at the best ways of achieving zinc adequacy later.) Zinc has a further role in helping the prostate, since it reduces the secretion of the substance prolactin, thereby increasing testosterone uptake by the prostate.

It has been shown that individuals with BPH, also have an imbalance in the quantities of, and ratios between, certain substances called essential fatty acids (EFA). There are a number of these extremely important nutrient factors (for details of sources, see pp. 59–60), but basically they can be divided into three groups: linoleic acid, linolenic acid and arachidonic acid. Correction of a deficiency in these, by nutritional alterations and supplementation, has been shown to dramatically improve the condition of individuals with BPH. (Results of trials involving this strategy will be given when EFA's are discussed in more detail, see pp. 57–60.)

The building blocks of protein are called amino acids, and there are over 20 of these. As mentioned previously, the use of a high protein diet can be helpful in normalizing the prostate (although there are other good reasons why a very high protein diet is not desirable long-term for many people). It has been found that three of the amino acids taken in combination — glycine, alinine and glutamic acid — are capable of dramatically improving BPH, and we will examine evidence of this, as well as the dosages recommended, in following chapters.

One of the greatest dangers accompanying BPH is that of a possible malignant change occurring. It has been noted that the breakdown products of cholesterol are cancer producing, and that these have a tendency to accumulate in the prostate gland when enlarged. For this reason, as well as for general health improvement, it is important for cholesterol levels to be maintained at safe limits. What these limits are and how to achieve them are discussed in a later chapter, but they do involve a reduction in sugar intake as well as ensuring an adequate fibre intake. There are other good reasons for a dietary pattern which includes a high fibre content, not the least being the need for bowel regularity. It has been shown that constipation is a frequent co-symptom with BPH and there is every chance that the long-term increase in pressure caused by constipation, as well as the tendency this produces for straining, are factors in the production of congestion in the lower pelvic region in which the prostate lies. Improvement in bowel function, through correct dietary practices, must be an element in any prostate self-help programme.

These in brief, then, are the nutrient strategies which are necessary for coping with existing prostate enlargement, as well as for preventing its occurrence in the first place. No one of these elements alone is sufficient; rather it is necessary to restructure the diet to provide adequate levels of protein, limit refined carbohydrate intake and ensure that zinc and its co-factors are adequately present, along with a correct quantity and balance of essential fatty acids. Specific amino acid combinations should also be added, and control exercised to maintain healthy cholesterol levels. All these should be combined with sufficient fibre intake to ensure a sound bowel function.

This may sound complicated, but fortunately the different components of this approach to correct an enlarged prostate are interacting, and so a basic dietary approach will take care of most of the requirements.

There are other elements which may be incorporated into a prostate gland health programme including extracts of pollen, which are noted as being helpful, as well as the use of ginseng and extracts of the fruit of the palm tree, Sereno Repens. These will be outlined briefly in subsequent chapters as adding to the overall value of the nutritional approach.

It is important that the programme presented in later chapters is followed in full, not just in part. There would doubtless be benefit derived from taking just one element, such as zinc, and hoping for an improvement. However, the various elements of the diet should be seen as interacting, and all should be used to achieve the greatest long-term benefit.

5.

Some Self-help Treatments

Structure and function are obviously interrelated and mutually interdependent. The way something is constructed determines the use to which it can be put (try cutting bread with a toothbrush); similarly the way something is used will alter its structure (even a sharp knife becomes dull with regular use). The human body is constructed to be used in a set number of ways. However if the body is incorrectly used, its shape and structure can be altered. For instance, posture can vary and alter with occupation and habitual use, and as the structure (posture) alters, the function of the component parts is forced to alter too. Take someone who is habitually stooped, their chest cage will be depressed rather than open, and their abdominal contents, the organs and structures of the digestive and reproductive systems, will be crowded. This produces alterations in the way these organs function, as well as increasing the degree of congestion in them.

In good body mechanics the chest is held high, the diaphragm (which separates the chest from the abdominal cavity) is also high, and the abdominal wall is flat and firm. When posture is poor and mechanics inferior, the chest is depressed, the diaphragm is unable to move adequately up and down with respiration, and the abdominal wall bulges out, as the contents of the abdominal cavity are pushed down towards the floor of the pelvis. This creates problems not just in the pelvic region and the prostate, of course; it can also cause the liver and stomach to alter their positions, as well as crowding of the intestinal canal. Functional changes take place in these regions as a consequence, and are often responsible for health problems, some of which can be quite serious. The drag of the organs on their supporting ligaments, for instance, can produce strains and tears such as occur in hiatus hernia, etc. The circulation of blood to, and through, these regions is dramatically altered in such a situation. The only source of drainage of blood, lymph, etc., from the pelvic organs, is via the abdominal veins, which are severely affected by distention of the abdominal contents downwards. These factors are thought by many eminent researchers to relate to the problems of bladder and prostate experienced by men, and to the malposition of the uterus in women, which can lead to period problems and pregnancy difficulties.

The nerve supply to these organs is also dependent upon sound body mechanics, involving the lower back and pelvic structures. Thus postural factors and the way the body is used are of importance in our assessment of causes of prostate dysfunction. Sagging abdominal contents; poorly functioning diaphragmatic movement in breathing; long periods of stasis when sitting, inadequate exercise and, as mentioned above, straining at stool, all add to the problems of the region in terms of poor circulation, poor nerve supply and poor drainage.

Congestion leads to altered nutritional status of the region, for no matter how good the diet, if the nutrients cannot adequately be transported, and the waste products adequately drained, the end result is an impoverished region with the potential for disease and poor function. This is the pattern in prostate hypertrophy in many men.

Sexual factors impinge upon this as well. When a man has intercourse, the following sequence of events occurs in the region of the prostate: initial stimulation, followed by erection, increases the prostate's secretion of fluids; with orgasm the seminal vesicles and the vas deferens contract, as do the ejaculatory ducts, and the sperm is delivered through the urethra; this is followed by relaxation of tension and dissipation of congestion in the region. However, sexual stimulation which is not followed by orgasm has many potentially deleterious effects, including inflammation of the urethra, local discomfort in the perineal area due to congestion, as well as possible impotence, and, as would be expected, prostate enlargement accompanying the chronic congestion resulting from this practice. In short, normal sexual practices are not damaging to a person's health, but interruption of the cycle leading to orgasm can be.

In general terms, then, the normalization of posture and regular exercise are to be encouraged. This may involve advice and/or treatment from a suitably qualified practitioner, such as an osteopath, to correct any faults in spinal and pelvic mechanics. Also, it is essential to avoid any straining over bowel movements, and to this end the dietary advice to be found later in the book will be of great assistance. However, using this knowledge of the link between structure and function, a number of effective self-treatments can be devised.

Hydrotherapy
A form of simple hydrotherapy can be extremely effective in reducing local congestion of the pelvic floor. There are two methods of hydrotherapy advocated in cases of hypertrophy of the prostate.

Method 1
The first method involves local irrigation using a cool saline solution. This is not an enema in the sense of attempting to enhance elimination via the bowel. Rather it is a means of applying a cold liquid to a congested area in order to stimulate drainage.

An enema bag, containing about a quart of

water, into which 2 teaspoons of salt have been dissolved, is required. The temperature of the water should have been reduced to about 55° to 60°F, by refrigeration. (Mix the salt with water, add to the bag and refrigerate until used.)

Bedtime is a good time to perform the local irrigation. The bowels should have been opened some time previously, so that the need for defecation is not current. Sitting upright on the toilet the patient introduces the tip of the application tube into the rectum, using a little lubricant on the tip for ease of entry. The enema bag with water should be suitably suspended nearby. It must of course be higher than the body of the individual, so that gravity will allow water to enter the rectum with ease.

The initial amount allowed into the rectum is about 4 fluid ounces (approximately $\frac{1}{2}$ a cup) of cold saline mixture. This is retained for about half a minute and then allowed to be expelled into the toilet bowl. This is followed after a minute or so of rest by the same procedure. Altogether the pattern is repeated 7 or 8 times which should use up the whole quart of water.

The method described produces an alternating hot and cold effect locally, within the rectum, and this closely approximates the prostate circulatory system. The cold applications cool the area down, and natural body heat warms it up again during the rest period between irrigations. This should be done three times weekly by anyone with BPH. Benefits will soon be noted and the practice may be reduced in frequency as improvement continues.

Method 2

A further measure which may be useful is the alternating immersion of the pelvis in hot and cold water. This is valuable because it not only gives relief to painful and distressing symptoms, but also helps to reduce congestion and to thus restore normal structure. It is especially helpful in relieving what is known as connective tissue stasis, an extreme congestion of the tissues, and is in this way a unique therapeutic agent.

Run about 5 inches of hot water (not hot enough to scald but as hot as is tolerable) into the bath and sit in this for a half to one minute. Alongside the bath should be a bowl sufficiently deep to allow for some 5 inches of cold water, and large enough to sit in — a large plastic bowl or an old-fashioned hip bath would do. (Years ago a proper portable bath was made for this purpose, which had a sloping back and a sitting arrangement so that the feet could rest comfortably on the floor whilst the pelvis was immersed.)

The idea of the bath is to sit, with the knees bent, so that the buttocks and the pelvic area (up to no higher than the navel) are covered with water. After the immersion in hot water transfer rapidly to the cold water for a further half to one minute, after which the pattern may be repeated once more, of hot followed by cold, for the same lengths of time.

If it is not possible to arrange a second bath or bowl for the cold immersion, then the water from the hot bath should be drained away and replaced with cold water. This delays the contrast element of the procedure somewhat, but is better than nothing.

Between immersions keep up the level of warmth by wrapping yourself in a towel, at the same time ensuring that the room itself is warm.

This alternation of hot and cold has a most beneficial effect on local circulation and may be performed daily if possible, or on alternate days, when the irrigation (Method 1) is not being used.

If it is not possible to alternate immersion in hot and cold water, hot and cold towels may be used instead to create a similar effect. For this a series of towels are wrung out in hot water and placed over the lower groin and lower back, and between the legs, ensuring the anus is well-covered. Repeated reapplications of hot towels to these regions are carried out over a fifteen to twenty minute period. The heat should be strong, but obviously not excessive enough to cause any discomfort in this sensitive region. Each towel should remain in position for a minute or two, before being replaced. After about fifteen minutes a cold application should be made in the same areas by wringing out towels in cold water. These should be applied quickly and left in place for a minute or so.

Exercise

Another important aid to improving the health of this part of the body is exercise. Bending and stretching are especially beneficial as this helps break down any congestion. Brisk walking everyday is also a good idea.

Yoga-type exercises in particular are helpful, and those which safely invert the body (the shoulder stand, for example, or the plough position) are highly recommended. Initially at least these should only be undertaken with the supervision of a qualified yoga instructor.

Some simple yoga postures which can be practised and are helpful in improving prostate drainage and circulation are outlined below.

The first is a very simple kneeling pose. This is easy to achieve unless there are problems with the knees and hips, in which case it should not be attempted. Before doing the postures, remove your shoes and any clothes that might be constricting. Make sure that the floor is not too hard — use a rug or a carpeted floor — and the room is warm.

Position 1
Sit on your heels, keeping your back straight. Breathe deeply and relax, then slowly allow your feet to separate so that your buttocks sink between them until they rest on the floor. Breathe deeply several times, allowing the muscles of the legs to relax completely as you breathe out. Keep the spine straight all the time. This has a stimulating effect on the circulation to the pelvic region and should be maintained for a minute or two. Repeat the position daily.

Position 2
The next pose is one which requires a little practice. Lie on your back on the floor (don't put a cushion under your head), then let the arms

extend sideways at an angle of about 45° to the rest of the body with the palms flat on the floor. Place the soles of your feet together, and draw the legs upwards, bending at the knees and allowing the weight of these to spread themselves apart as the soles are brought higher. As you lift your legs, your buttocks will ease off the floor. This is the upper limit of the pose and should be held for a minute or so. Breathe deeply and slowly all the while, until you feel you wish to roll back downwards to lie flat on the floor. If it is difficult to maintain the position once the buttocks have left the floor, place a small cushion under the buttocks to help to support the position.

In this position of inverted gravity (i.e. the pelvic organs are hanging upside down, so to speak) and with the legs spread as they should be, there is a release of pressure on the pelvic floor which benefits the prostate. This posture should be done daily.

Position 3
This is an alternative to position 2. Kneel on the floor with your weight on your knees and hands. Allow your arms to bend until your forehead rests on the floor and your buttocks are in the air. In this position — which once again inverts the internal organs and releases pressure from the pelvic floor — breathe deeply and at the same time retract your abdomen, i.e. pull your tummy in and up, as though the umbilicus (navel) is being drawn towards the spine. Hold this position and your breath for a few seconds, then release your breath and allow your

abdomen to relax again. Repeat this ten times. When you have completed the exercise, sit for a while on your haunches before rising, as you may feel dizzy. (This is true of all floor exercises, especially if accompanied by deep breathing.) Please note: anyone with glaucoma or high blood pressure should avoid this posture until advice is sought from an expert as to their desirability.

These methods are suggested as part of a general attempt to improve abdominal muscle tone and pelvic circulation. There are many other yoga poses, and these may be studied from books or by attending classes.

Prostate Self-help with Reflex Pressure Points
Osteopathic research has shown that certain areas of the body's surface can be felt to change in texture, and to become sensitive to pressure, in response to various problems of the internal organs. When the prostate is disturbed there are two main reflex areas which become sensitive in this way. The first is an area on the outer thigh, about a third of the way between the hip and the knee which will usually be found to be tight. It has been described as feeling like an 'ensheathing callus'. When this is found (it may extend for some 6 inches or more in this region) and is sensitive to moderate pressure, it probably indicates lymphatic congestion of the prostate. (In women the same area is found to be related to uterine dysfunction.) It is possible to confirm the likelihood of this being an active reflex by also palpating the second area which is at the very base of the spine, between the prominent pelvic bone which lies just to the side

of the last vertebrae of the spine, and the spine itself. An area which feels tight and sensitive in this region, and which is also accompanied by the sensitive area on the outer thigh, is a confirmation of some reflex activity from the prostate (or uterus). These areas or points are known as Chapman's reflexes, after the osteopathic physician who charted them in the 1930s, or as neurolymphatic reflexes. (See Fig 4.)

Treatment of these points or areas involves the application of a moderate pressure first to the leg area, and then to the back area. A period of about 20 seconds of thumb pressure should be given at the tenderest part of the reflex area on the legs. Both legs should be treated in this way if both are found to contain tender reflex points in this region. This should be followed by a similar period of pressure on the reflex areas on the back (both sides of the spine if they are both tender to pressure).

It has been shown that the effect of this application of pressure is to reduce the lymphatic congestion in whichever area the points relate to, in this instance to the prostate gland. Lymphatic congestion indicates that circulation and drainage of the area is inadequate, and that there may be inflammation. Obviously this reflex stimulus will not cure the condition, but it will certainly help to reduce local swelling and may instigate symptomatic relief of the condition, at least for a while. This should therefore be seen as a method by which a degree of first aid may be given while long-term measures (such as diet) are being used.

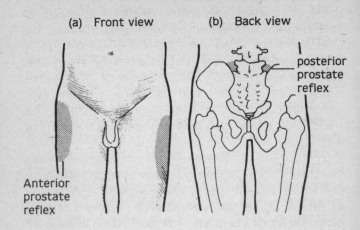

Fig 4   Neurolymphatic (Chapman's) reflexes

In order to avoid irritating the local tissues this method should not be applied more than once daily, and only when the reflex area is found to be sensitive. Doing more will not achieve better results, as it is possible to both exhaust a reflex and to irritate it. If it is found to be difficult to press on the points at the side of the base of the spine, then lying on the floor and placing a golf (or tennis) ball strategically under the point will allow for the appropriate degree of pressure to be applied.

This method can also be seen to be diagnostic and prognostic (telling you how the condition is progressing), since if lymphatic drainage improves (using the hydrotherapy methods and diet, etc) then these reflexes will no longer feel tender. (For a deeper understanding of neurolymphatic reflexes as they affect other parts of the body, my book *Soft Tissue Manipulation* should be consulted.)

Structure and function are inextricably linked, and we must use both, via these methods, to enhance the health of the region as a whole, and the prostate in particular. It is to be hoped that the methods discussed, especially the hydro-therapy measures, are not skipped over as being quaint relics of the past. There is ample evidence of their effectiveness, sometimes dramatically so. This effectiveness should never, however, be seen as being sufficient to allow the nutritional measures which are presented in the following chapters to be ignored. The nutritional aspect of prostate problems is the key to recovery.

6.

Zinc and the Prostate

Zinc is arguably the single most important element in any approach aimed at improving the condition of the prostate. A major study was undertaken in the USA on the relationship between zinc and the health of the prostate gland, and its findings were reported to the American Medical Association in 1974. The first element of the study involved assessing the presence of zinc in various tissues of the body. Some 750 patients were involved in the trials. Samples of blood were obtained and these were analysed, and the zinc levels determined. Samples of semen were examined and again zinc levels determined. Finally prostatic tissue itself was obtained, and zinc levels in these structures established.

The results confirmed that determination of zinc levels by the methods used was reliable, and that the results could be reproduced. The level of zinc found in the sperm was found to be a good indicator of the level of zinc concentration found in the prostate gland; this is important since it is not desirable to have to remove small parts of the gland in order to assess the zinc status of the person. Sperm evaluation proved to be just as accurate as evaluation of the actual tissues of the gland.

The overall results of the study of tissues showed that nearly 40 per cent of the males involved had borderline, or actual, zinc deficiency in the prostate. Those patients who had chronic prostatitis were almost inevitably low in zinc, in both the prostate and sperm analysis, and yet showed normal blood levels of the mineral. A supplement of zinc taken for between 2 and 16 weeks produced symptomatic relief in 70 per cent of the patients. The levels of zinc in the tissues discussed were shown to rise steadily while patients were on supplements.

In patients with cancer of the prostate there was again evidence of zinc deficiency in both sperm and the gland. When there was widespread dissemination of the cancer, the level of zinc in the blood was also shown to be low, but otherwise blood samples showed normal levels of zinc. This indicates that under usual conditions the assessment of zinc by taking a sample of blood is meaningless, insofar as the amounts present in the prostate structures and tissues is concerned.

In cases of prostate enlargement (BPH), where the size of the gland can increase from walnut size to the size of a medium orange, the blood levels were again shown to be normal as far as zinc was concerned, even when local tissues showed a deficit. When supplementation of zinc was carried out in BPH patients the serum levels stayed much the same, but the concentrations in the prostate and sperm increased markedly. These patients also displayed long-term improvement in their condition, as assessed by symptoms being reduced. There was observable shrinkage of the prostate, as assessed by palpation, X-ray examination, and direct observation using an endoscope, in the majority of these patients.

The report on these studies concludes thus:

Zinc may play a specific role in the pathophysiology and treatment of genitourinary diseases. Although zinc has been used as a therapeutic agent in wound healing, chronic ulcers, burns and hepatitis, it has not previously been utilized in a systematic manner, specifically for prostatic diseases.

And yet others had noted many of these findings previously; indeed the connection between prostate and zinc has been known for half a century or more. As Dr Carl Pfeiffer points out, in his classic book, *Mental and Elemental Nutrients*. 'Zinc is important for the formation of active sperm in all mammalian species, including man. The prostate and the prostatic secretions are high in zinc.' Dr Pfeiffer also points out that where inflammation of the prostate (prostatitis) exists the local zinc levels often drop to as low as one-tenth of normal levels.

Dr Irving Bush, of the Center for Studies of

Prostate Diseases, found that zinc supplementation abolished symptoms in the majority of men suffering from non-infective chronic prostatitis. Dr Kurt Donsbach of California has stated: 'A diseased prostate gland has a very low concentration of zinc, and for some reason vitamin C seems to be more potent, as an anti-infective agent, in the presence of zinc.' (We shall be considering the role of vitamin C later.)

The question obviously is how can we increase zinc levels through diet. Or in other words which foods contain significant amounts of zinc. This is important since it is patently undesirable to have to take large doses of any substance for unlimited, or very long periods, although in the short term this is probably the only way of boosting levels speedily.

The main food sources are as follows:

Milligrams of zinc per 100 grams (3 ounces) of food

Peas	4.0
Carrots	2.0
Beets	0.93
Cabbage	0.80
Oysters	143.0
Herrings	100.0
Clams	20.0
Wheat bran	14.0
Whole oatmeal	14.0
Brown rice	2.5
Dates	0.34
Bananas	0.28
Nuts	3.0
Whole wheat	1.04
Refined wheat	0.12

Egg	1.2
Cow's milk	Between 17 and 66
Human milk	Between 2 and 138
Human colostrum (present in first feed to the baby)	Between 70 and 900+
Pumpkin seeds, Sunflower seeds	Over 25

It is interesting to note the large variables in mothers' milk. Researchers such as Dr Pfeiffer suggest zinc supplementation for expectant mothers, since the first feed from the mother containing the colostrum should have a high level of zinc to counteract the high levels of copper with which a baby is born. It has even been suggested that the first seeds of later prostate trouble are sown shortly after birth, if the mother is low in zinc, or if no breast feeding occurs.

The daily requirement of zinc, in normal health, is around 15 milligrams. However it is important to remember that daily requirements vary from person to person. Some nutrients are required in greater quantities by one individual as compared to another, and these differences need not be small but may vary by a factor of 7 or more. Thus one person may require 10 to 15 milligrams of zinc daily, in order to remain healthy, and another may require 50 to 100 milligrams of the same nutrient. These differences are inborn and cannot be changed, or unfortunately easily recognized until problems arise in those who have great needs which are not being met.

We also require more zinc in different circumstances. For example during periods of rapid growth, during puberty, during pregnancy, during all periods of stress and infection, in response to frequent sex (or masturbation). In all such cases the body requires more zinc than normal. In order to utilize the zinc which is present, the body requires all other nutrients in a balanced form. Specifically zinc interacts with certain nutrients such as vitamin A, calcium, phosphorus and vitamin C, and is better utilized when these are present in adequate quantities. In particular, zinc has a relationship with a B vitamin called pyridoxine, (formerly known as vitamin B6). If zinc is taken as a supplement, as suggested later, it is important that there are sufficient levels of vitamin B6 and other nutrients for the zinc to be able to produce beneficial effects.

What can zinc do for the prostate and for sexual function? Pfeiffer puts it thus:

Zinc will do many things to lubricate the sexual machinery, such as,

1. Increase penis and testes size in young growing males;
2. Increase sperm motility;
3. Decrease prostatitis and normalize secretions;
4. Replace the zinc loss occasioned by excessive prostate secretion as in sexual foreplay, and replace the zinc lost in the ejaculate.
5. Help prevent impotency.

However he cautions that: 'With all this

knowledge we still cannot say that anyone's sex life would be better with excess zinc; we can only say that zinc is needed for normal sex activity, normal reproduction, and the perfection of babies of all species.'

Not only men need zinc, of course, for as indicated it is a vital element in breast milk, and is used by the body in large amounts during pregnancy. Pfeiffer points out that it is a vital factor in the health and production of the ova (the female egg). Vaginal secretions are also high in zinc.

Thus the tradition of eating oysters for fertility and sexual health is seen to be well founded in respect of their zinc content. Consumption of pumpkins seeds is a cheaper way of achieving a similar effect. Dr Donsbach states: 'Folk medicine in many countries of Europe tells us that the men of Bulgaria, Ukraine and Turkey were well aware of the fact that eating a handful of pumpkin seeds daily would prevent prostate problems, and thus enhance their virility.' It is suggested that such seeds contain not only abundant zinc, but other substances, including plant hormones, which benefit man. They also contain desirable forms of essential fatty acids, which we will consider later.

The best forms of zinc to take as a supplement are thought to be zinc orotate or zinc picolinate. This combines the zinc with a substance called orotic acid, which aids its absorption and transportation. Tablets of zinc orotate are in strengths of 100 milligrams (see pp. 49–50 for sources). This is not all zinc, though, for that would represent an excessive intake. Rather it is about 15 per cent zinc and the rest is is orotic acid. This provides the daily intake requirement with each tablet, and together with a good supply of zinc from selected foods, as mentioned above, this should replenish stocks of zinc rapidly. As an alternative to zinc orotate 50 milligrams daily of zinc picolinate may be taken.

One note of caution: excessive zinc intake competes in the gut for absorption with iron and copper, and long-term zinc supplementation might decrease levels of these important substances. Thus supplementation should be carried out every other day or on 5 or 6 days weekly, ideally at the same time as ensuring an abundant supply of zinc from food such as sunflower and pumpkin seeds, herrings, etc. The nutrients vitamin B6 and vitamin C should be taken as well and the correct doses of these will be given later in the book. Although the importance of zinc is indisputable, it is essential that other nutrients are not neglected.

7.

Fats and Essential Fatty Acids: Their Effects on the Prostate

Modern man consumes a phenomenal amount of fat. Unfortunately this fat is largely made up of a type of fat, called saturated fat, which is considered to be highly detrimental to health. The type of meat eaten and the amount of dairy produce consumed seem to be largely responsible for this, and the role these elements have played in man's diet has changed dramatically in the past century (as, incidentally, has the incidence of prostate hypertrophy and prostate cancer). Another factor which has altered is the way in which animals are reared for consumption. The trend until recently has been for a far higher fat content, although growing awareness seems now to be leading away from this trend.

Leading health authorities, world wide, have told us that no more than 30 per cent of our total energy intake should be derived from fats, and that no more than half of this should be in the form of saturated fats. At present the intake of fats in the Western world is around 40 per cent of total energy consumption, and the ratio between saturated and polyunsaturated fats (the more desirable type) shows that in the UK we eat nearly four times as much saturated as unsaturated fat (instead of equal amounts).

The consequences for health and disease of all this is very important indeed, relating as it does to coronary heart disease, diabetes, gall bladder disease and cancer. It also relates to prostate problems. In primitive times fat consumption was around 20 per cent of total energy intake, and even the type of fat consumed was different, since free-living animals (game) contain only about 4 per cent of their total body weight as fat (most of this being unsaturated fat) as compared to some 30 per cent of body weight comprising fat in modern beef cattle (and most of this being saturated fat). These are the changes which have contributed to the epidemic proportions of some of the diseases mentioned, as well as to prostate disease.

As mentioned previously we share prostate problems with our close friend the dog. Experiments in the USA, at Rutgers University, showed that elderly dogs with prostate problems could be helped considerably, with reduction in the size of the prostate, by reducing the cholesterol levels in their blood. Cholesterol levels in the body relate to both a high saturated fat and a high sugar content of the diet.

Examination of human prostates after death,

in 100 men with BPH, showed that these glands contained 80 per cent more cholesterol on average than normal prostate glands.

Observation in rural Africa shows that people on a low fat diet had low prostate risk. When the same people changed to a Western dietary pattern, with a high fat (and sugar) content, the production of hormones associated with high incidence of prostate problems rose dramatically.

When similar trials were carried out in reverse, in the USA, white males with a normally high fat intake and associated production of undesirably high levels of these hormones, were shown to reverse this trend when placed, for just a matter of weeks, on a low fat diet. This was seen as evidence of a reduced risk of prostate cancer in the men whose diet was low in fat.

In order to reduce the incidence of prostate enlargement and specifically of prostate cancer, there should be a major effort directed at reducing both fat intake, altering fat type, and in reducing sugar intake. All of these factors are interrelated in the development of high cholesterol levels in the blood, and ultimately in the prostate. This calls for a reduction in the eating of meat derived from domesticated farmed animals such as cattle, pig, sheep, etc. It also means avoiding fried food and the skin on chicken. Dairy produce such as milk, full fat cheese and butter also come under suspicion and should be reduced drastically.

This leaves fish, poultry (apart from the skin), low fat dairy produce, such as skimmed milk, low fat cheese such as feta and edam, and low fat yoghurt (margarines which are not high in polyunsaturated fats and butter, however should be avoided), meat as long as it is game, (such as rabbit, hare, deer), vegetables, fruit, grains, pulses — all of which would be included in a healthy diet.

However, it has been shown, as previously commented, that sugar also increases cholesterol levels in the blood, and so consumption of this should be reduced to minimal levels too. No white or brown sugar products should be eaten, including cakes, sweets, pastries as well as sugar itself, if prostate problems are to be avoided. We obtain ample natural sugar from our fruit and vegetable intake and the refined sugars present in so many foods are harmful in a number of respects, not least being the promotion of heart problems, cancer and obesity.

A diet rich in fibre is a must. Fibre is best obtained simply by eating abundant vegetables and fruits, as well as foods derived from the pulse family (lentils, chickpeas, beans, etc).

The combination of a diet low in saturated fats, high in fibre, and low in sugar is the key to health in general and prostate health in particular.

In addition we must ensure an adequate intake of those fats which are useful, the essential fatty acids. These have a beneficial effect on the prostate and on health in general.

Essential Fatty Acids and the Prostate
In the early 1940s two doctors in California

noticed that some of the patients to whom they were giving high dosages of vitamin F (another name for essential fatty acids or EFA) were showing marked improvements in the status of their enlarged prostates. Drs Hart and Cooper went on to conduct a clinical trial on some 20 patients using this approach. This is what they did. They palpated the size of the enlarged prostate of each participant in the trial; took a sample of urine as well as a detailed record of symptoms such as urinary problems, including weakness of the urine stream, dribbling, passing water during the night and cystitis (bladder inflammation). The patients were all given thorough investigations to exclude the possibility of other factors such as hormone or nutrient imbalances. Blood samples were taken to note the various levels of fats and other substances. Hormone levels were monitored and the patients were then placed on vitamin F (essential fatty acid) supplementation.

Re-examination was carried out at monthly intervals at which time all procedures, as described above, were repeated. The patients also reported weekly on any changes which they had noted.

The results were very impressive indeed. All cases showed a reduction in the amount of urine left in the bladder after the individual had passed water. This residual urine makes the bladder prone to infection as the stagnant urine is an ideal medium for bacteria. In 12 out of the 19 patients who completed the trial there was a complete absence of residual urine at the end of the treatment period, and consequently an absence of previously noted cystitis. In 13 of the cases there was elimination of the need to pass water during the night. There was, in all patients, a decrease in fatigue and leg pains, as well as an increase in sexual interest. Dribbling was eliminated in 18 of the 19 patients, and the force of the urine stream increased. In all cases there was a rapid reduction in the size of the prostate, confirmed by palpation.

All the patients showed enthusiasm over the improvement in their physical well-being. Those that showed less improvement than the others had all had a history of gonorrhoeal infection in the past.

The beneficial effects of the essential fatty acids do not stop with the prostate. They aid in preventing cholesterol deposits forming in the arteries; they promote healthy skin and hair; they protect against the harmful effects of X-rays; they improve and support glandular function and help to ensure calcium availability to cells; they combat cardiovascular disease and assist in the burning (metabolizing) of saturated fats, thus reducing their harmful potential and assisting in weight reduction.

There are numerous safe sources of essential fatty acids. Among the best of these are linseed oil (flax seed), sunflower and pumpkin seeds. EFA are also plentiful in walnuts, almonds, pecan nuts and avocado pears (note that brazil and cashew nuts do not have a high level of EFA). Eating a fresh salad every day garnished with sunflower seeds and fresh nuts, or sprinkling linseed on to a bowl of cereal will supply an adequate amount of EFA to your diet.

The body can manufacture the other essential fatty acids if sufficient linoleic acid, which is found in a wide range of foods, including vegetables and grains, is present.

Apart from adding foods high in these oils to the diet, it is possible to obtain them by taking supplements specifically formulated to supply the right quantities and types of fatty acids. It is advisable to take such supplements with vitamin E, in supplement form, and to do so at mealtimes. It is also important to be aware that the more carbohydrate consumed, the more essential fatty acids the body requires. A daily supplement of linseed oil (be sure to obtain a form which is designed for human consumption) at a rate of 1 to 2 tablespoons of the oil daily is recommended. Evening Primrose oil is available in health food stores. This is an excellent if slightly expensive way of obtaining EFA's and 500 to 1,000 milligrams daily (one or two capsules) of this should be taken. On the other hand an inexpensive way of obtaining adequate supplies is to eat a handful of pumpkin and/or sunflower seeds, twice daily.

By avoiding excessive saturated fat (meat, dairy products, etc) and sugars, and by ensuring adequate intake of EFA's as laid out here, a major contribution will be made to general health and to prostate well-being.

We will now consider other nutrients and substances, such as pollen and ginseng, as well as the role of protein and particular amino acids in the prevention and safe treatment of prostate problems.

8.

Nutrient Therapies for Prostate Problems

We have already seen that there is strong evidence that a high protein diet acts as a protective agent against prostate enlargement. As with most of the body's structures the cells which compose the prostate gland are largely constructed of protein. Cells of glandular structures, however, have a uniquely high protein component. This is one reason why these are often the parts of animals which are eaten first, from choice, by predators and by primitive hunter-gatherer people. Such people choose to eat the organs such as the spleen, liver and glands, before bothering to eat the muscle meats which are so much the dominant choice of Western man. Predators make similar choices, leaving the muscle meat to last, or to scavenging animals such as hyenas and vultures.

The ratios of the various building blocks of protein which make up the particular cells of different glands varies, as would be expected, thus imparting the unique characteristics of each gland or organ. It is conceivable that a very high protein diet (44 per cent protein, 35 per cent carbohydrate, 21 per cent fat), provides the particular amino acids needed to protect the health of the prostate. This type of diet is close to that followed by hunter-gatherer people, who also consume large amounts of plant food, and thus avoid the over-acidification of the body which could result from excessive protein intake.

An alternative to the consumption of huge amounts of protein is, however, readily available. This involves supplementing the diet with three specific amino acids (out of the twenty odd there are in total), in order to achieve amazing benefits to enlarged prostate conditions.

A report appeared as long ago as 1958, in the *Journal of the Maine Medical Association*, which described an important trial using these three amino acids, glycine, alanine and glutamic acid, in combination. The trial involved 45 men who all had BPH with a range of symptoms which included discomfort, night-time urgency, delayed urination (an inability to begin to pass water when this was desired), frequency of urination and uncontrollable urgency. These patients varied in age from 37 to 75, and most had had the complaint for at least 4 years. Half of the men were given the supplement of amino acids and the other half received a placebo (a dummy tablet). The tablets were taken after meals for three months.

The results were startling. Of those who had received the real amino acid tablets, over 90 per cent were found to have a reduction in size of the prostate, and in a third, the prostate had returned to normal size. The need to pass water at night was totally eliminated in three-quarters of these patients, with over 90 per cent reporting a marked improvement in this symptom. Urgency was relieved in 80 per cent of these patients and almost the same percentage lost the frequency symptoms, with 70 per cent noting absence of the symptom of delayed urination.

Those who had been given the dummy tablets showed no such improvement until they were eventually placed on the amino acid supplementation.

Since there is no danger at all from supplementation using a natural substance, such as an amino acid, in the dosages used, this was an extremely successful result. Interestingly a number of other symptoms, including tendency to swellings in various parts of the body, improved at the same time. This symptom is characteristic of protein deficiency which might well have been the underlying cause, alleviated by the amino acid therapy.

Suggested dosages are: glycine–200 mg per day; glutamic acid — 200 mg per day; and alinine — 200 mg per day.

Amino acids and nutrients such as zinc orotate are available from Cantassium Co., 225 Putney Bridge Road, London SW15 2PY, and from Nature's Best Health Products, PO Box 1, Tunbridge Wells, Kent, TN2 3EQ.

Pollen and the Prostate

Pollen is rich both in protein and essential fatty acids, and of course in plant hormones, so the benefits found from its use in treating a number of conditions, including prostate enlargement, may be related to the presence of any one of these constituents, or to all of them.

A report appeared in the *Swedish Medical Journal* in 1961, describing the use of pollen extract tablets manufactured by the firm B. Cernelle. Out of ten patients with BPH five were relieved of their symptoms and the prostate size returned to normal over a one-year treatment period. The patients with inflamed prostates showed a most marked improvement.

A Japanese trial at Nagasaki University School of Medicine, Department of Urology, used the same pollen extracts on some 30 patients, all suffering from acute prostatitis. The results showed that just over half of the patients, 16 in all, enjoyed results described as 'markedly effective'. Another 13 cases were 'effective', but not as strongly so, and in only one case was there no improvement.

In the Swedish trial four tablets of pollen (named 'Cernilton') were taken daily, and in the Japanese trials a higher intake of six tablets daily was used. In none of the trials was there any report of side-effects.

It seems likely that the combination of fatty acids, plant hormones and protein present in pollen was responsible for the benefits noted in these two trials.

Another plant used in the treatment of the prostate, and in other conditions, is ginseng.

Ginseng and Prostate Problems

Long employed as an aphrodisiac and general tonic in the Orient, ginseng (*Panax* ginseng) is the powdered root of this remarkable plant. It is known to contain a number of properties, one of which enhances the male hormone testosterone. It also decreases prostate weight when administered regularly.

In those suffering from BPH there is a decreased level of testosterone, with a corresponding drop in the intestinal absorption of zinc. A vicious cycle results which ends ultimately in enlargement of the gland. Ginseng used regularly would appear to provide benefits in terms of all of these negative factors. No clinical trials have been reported, but there is a long tradition of the successful use of ginseng in the Orient and in individual patients in the West. It would seem to provide a useful supportive role whilst more fundamental action is being taken, through the use of added essential fatty acids and zinc, for example.

20 drops of the fluid extract of ginseng are taken three times daily as a therapeutic dose. It is important that genuine *Panax* ginseng is obtained as the demand for this substance has led to a plethora of inferior products reaching the market.

Russian research in particular has resulted in a degree of respectability being granted to the use of ginseng and other remarkable plant substances, like the Siberian eleutherococcus. Such plant substances are known as adaptogens, and are believed to be able to increase the general capacity of the body to overcome external stresses through adaptation. This has implications relating to the ageing process as well as to factors such as radiation damage (which is in itself an acceleration of the ageing process).

One of the key benefits of adaptogens is that they can enhance the body's ability to utilize oxygen. This in itself is a crucial factor in terms of the ageing process, and therefore is part of the complex of factors negatively affecting prostate function as a man gets older.

All adaptogens work slowly; they do not produce sudden changes, but have to be used for some weeks before any noticeable alteration in symptoms will be felt. Eleutherococcus is at least as powerful an adaptogen as ginseng and these two substances are available generally. However their popularity has led to cheap imitations being placed on the market, and it is important that only active forms are used. Check sources carefully to ensure that only genuine *Panax* ginseng or Siberian eleutherococcus are used. Health food stores should be able to guide you as to the quality of the adaptogen of your choice.

It is also worth remembering that the use of adaptogens should be seen as just one part of a general approach which includes the nutritional advice already presented. Adaptogens on their own will not produce a complete reversal of a change which involves deficits of crucial nutrients, such as zinc and essential fatty acids.

Sereno Repens
The fruit of the palm tree (saw palmetto

berries, also known as *sabal serrulata*) contains substances which inhibit various biochemical activities related to the development of BPH. Their action leads to a reduction in the activity of 5-alpha reductase which trials in humans and animals have shown to be effective in aiding reduction in the size of the prostate gland in BPH.

20 drops of the fluid extract of this plant's berries are taken three times daily as a therapeutic dose. Again this should be accompanied by the use of nutritional support in the way of protein, essential fatty acids and zinc.

Raw Glandular Extracts and the Prostate

Over the past fifty years or more a science has grown around the use of extracts of glandular substances derived from healthy young animals. These glands secrete hormonal substances in the animal, and they are remarkably similar to the glands found in humans. It has been found that depending upon the method of extraction and preservation of such glandular substances, they can have a profound effect on the human body, by supplying it with the essential raw materials contained within the glands. The body is able to utilize these to its benefit in many conditions, including prostate enlargement.

The glands which interact within what is known as the endocrine system, include the pituitary, thymus, pineal, hypothalamus, thyroid and parathyroid, adrenals, kidney, pancreas and the gonads or sex glands. Imbalances between hormones occur, and other secretions from these various glands become deficient and unbalanced as a consequence of age or ill-health, and especially if there is a lack of balanced nutritional pattern. It is the rebalancing of these secretions which the use of glandular extracts is designed to achieve.

The most potent method of achieving effects is by injecting such glandular substances. This process often receives publicity when notable personalities are reported as having 'youth enhancing' therapy via glandular treatment. It is the chance of a degree of youthful regeneration and vitality which has made this such a fashionable and expensive process. However a much less expensive, if moderately less effective, method exists which involves taking glandular extracts orally in tablet or capsule form. It used to be thought that this route was useless, since the digestive process would reduce any hormone or enzyme molecules present into their constituent amino acids, thus making them no more therapeutic than a piece of cheese or an egg. However, recent research has shown that the claims of the endocrinologists, advocating oral use of glandular substances, were not far fetched, since around half of large molecule substances such as enzymes pass through the digestive process intact. It is also now known that a good proportion of these will reach the tissues of the body intact, as complex proteins. Thus it is noted that such elements of the original tissue, whether hormone, enzyme, polypeptide, essential fatty acid, etc, can and do reach appropriate tissues and can therefore aid in their regeneration and health enhancement.

The most used of these substances is the extract of thymus gland, which has an effect on the total immune function (defence system) of the body, and which influences all other glandular centres in the body. Other tissues are now being used in therapeutic settings, and where appropriate some, such as liver, stomach, heart, etc, are being provided in tablet form. Sometimes a general mixture of all the available tissues is given, in a sort of cocktail which the body can then sort out as its needs dictate. Such a mixture, together with an extract of prostate and/or orchic tissue (testicles), is used in prostate regeneration treatment. It has been found that these are better utilized when a sound general nutritional status exists, and so they should be seen as a part of a general approach, rather than as remedies on their own.

Research has shown that the method of extraction of these glandular substances is critical to their potential value. The methods used include freeze drying, heat processing and salt precipitation. Without going into technical detail it is apparent to researchers that freeze drying results in the maximum retention of vital elements. It also avoids removal of the fat content, which is vital for the maintenance of some of the fat-soluble enzymes in these tissues. Another key element in the value of the extract is the source of the animal which has been used to provide the extract. Those exposed to insecticides and hormone treatment will be substandard compared to those not so contaminated. In general it is considered that the extracts derived from New Zealand animals are safer than others. Glandulars which are 'buffered' are more likely to pass through the initial stages of digestion unscathed, and thus be available for uptake by the body and transportation to the desired site.

Prostate and male glandular formula are available from Larkhall Laboratories, 225 Putney Bridge Road, London SW15 2PY and prostate tissue concentrate, as well as prostate and orchic concentrate, are available from Nature's Best Health Products, PO Box 1, Tunbridge Wells, Kent, TN2 3EQ. Many health food stores also carry supplies of glandular extracts or 'raw' glandulars, and it is desirable that sources and methods of manufacture be assessed before the purchase and use of these substances. The reason for taking orchic tissues relates to the fact that one of the major roles of the testes is to produce testosterone, the hormone which maintains prostate health and size, and which, if deficient, results in enlargement. It is thus desirable that testicular function be enhanced, as well as prostate. If such glandular extracts are taken, it is important that adequate essential fatty acid intake and zinc also be included in the programme, as discussed in chapter 4.

A normal course of treatment for the use of glandular substances is six weeks, with two tablets of prostate extract being taken after each meal. The course can be repeated after a two month interval, if still required.

Summary of Nutrient Supplements

- Zinc — as an orotate or picolinate: if Zinc orotate is taken, the dose is 100 to 200 milligrams daily for five or six days per week, and one tablet of chelated copper on alternate days; if Zinc picolinate is taken, then dosage is 50 milligrams daily for six days per week for at least six months. Chelated copper should be taken on alternate days (providing one milligram of copper). Also, 50 to 100 milligrams of vitamin B6 should be taken daily.
- Fatty acid supplementation — take 1 tablespoon of linseed oil twice daily and/or two 500 milligram capsules of Oil of Evening Primrose. Also, vitamin E, 200 to 400 iu should be taken daily, with EFA supplements.
- Amino acids — Glycine, alanine and glutamic acid, take 200 milligrams of each daily together.
- Pollen extract — Cernilton tablets, take three to six tablets daily.
- Sereno repens — 20 drops of fluid extract to be taken three times daily.
- Panax ginseng — 20 drops of fluid extract to be taken three times daily.
- Raw glandular extracts — prostate and orchic, 2 tablets after each meal for six weeks, every three months.

In all of these measures a period of not less than six months should be considered as a basic time scale. After this, if results have been satisfactory, a maintenence dosage of zinc and essential fatty acids, of about 25 per cent of the therapeutic doses given above, is suggested indefinitely.

The nutrients and other substances discussed above are all related to BPH and to prostatitis. One of the major accompanying problems of these conditions is frequent cystitis and urethritis. In order to improve this a major contribution can be achieved from the judicious use of vitamin C.

Vitamin C's Role in Prostate Problems, Cystitis and Urethritis

It is reported by authorities in the USA that effective treatment of urethritis (inflammation of the tube carrying the urine and sperm out of the body) can be achieved by taking 3 grams of vitamin C daily for four days.

When there is retention of urine, so common in prostate enlargement, there is a danger of infection and inflammation of the bladder. Chronic cystitis (inflammation of the bladder) can result from decomposition of the ammonia in the urine in such a situation. This increases the tendency for the urine to become more alkaline and less acid, which in turn can result in crystals forming in the urine, causing pain and irritation. The increased acidity in the urine which accompanies high doses of some forms of vitamin C (ascorbic acid) helps to reverse this tendency, relieving the symptoms rapidly and reducing the dangers of infection. Some people take as much as 10 grams of vitamin C daily when cystitis is common, and this achieves the desired results quickly, and avoids the dangers of kidney infection (pyelitis) which can result from infection in the urinary tract.

Linus Pauling, the double Nobel prizewinner

and advocate of vitamin C in therapy, maintains that when large amounts of vitamin C are taken as much as 60 per cent of the substance which reaches the blood stream, ends up being voided in the urine. This though is not a waste, by any means, because of the benefits it brings to the urinary tract (bladder, urethra, etc). Pauling also claims that taking vitamin C can dramatically reduce the dangers of bladder cancer.

As mentioned in an earlier chapter vitamin C acts as an anti-infection agent far more efficiently when it is in the presence of adequate zinc. It thus makes sense that in attempting to normalize prostate problems, including the side effects of prostate enlargement, urethritis and cystitis, vitamin C should be a major element in the treatment programme.

Between 1 and 3 grams of vitamin C should be taken daily in separate doses, during the therapeutic period (six months at least) and if there is an active inflammation of the urethra or bladder this can be increased to as much as 10 grams per day until symptoms decrease. This high dosage of vitamin C could result in diarrhoea, which will rapidly be relieved when the vitamin C dose is reduced a little. It is a minor inconvenience, however, compared with the side effects of drugs commonly used in treating such conditions (see also next chapter).

In Chapter 10 we consider a dietary pattern which should accompany this type of nutrient therapy. The diet is of course a fundamental source of many of the nutrients discussed and so should be seen as an ongoing concern, not something to use for a while and then abandon. The problems of the prostate are the result of years of wrong eating among other factors, and the reform of the diet is therefore a basic requirement of prostate health.

The objectives of such a diet should be to comprehensively deal with the provision of the various nutrients already discussed, as well as promoting other factors such as bowel health and cholesterol normality, via a high fibre content.

9.

Inflammation of the Prostate: Causes and Treatment

The major consideration so far has been enlargement of the prostate (BPH) and its consequences. In passing we have looked at some of the methods in which an inflamed or infected prostate (prostatitis) might be helped, but now we will concentrate on this aspect of the problem, since it represents a more aggravating development than simple enlargement.

As has already been shown there are a number of ways in which inflammation and/or infection can arise. These include the development of crystals of phosphate in the urethra and bladder due to inadequate acidification of the urine. Another cause is the development of bacterial activity in stagnant urine, when the bladder is unable to be emptied efficiently. This is often combined with decomposition of the ammonia in the bladder urine. There may be primary infection elsewhere, such as in the teeth. Organisms may multiply in prostatic fluid itself, which normally contains antibacterial elements, but which may not be thus protected at this time because of inadequate nutrient status involving zinc, essential fatty acids and probably vitamin C. There are other forms of crystaline development which may occur if the urine is excessively acidic.

The Prostate and Recurrent Urinary Infections
The questionnaire on pp. 20–21 outlines the commonest indicators of prostate enlargement (benign prostatic hypertrophy). There is one other sign which should lead to suspicion of prostate enlargement, and this is recurrent urinary tract infections.

If a relapse occurs after appropriate antibiotic therapy then this may indicate a number of possibilities. Among these are kidney infection, a stone obstructing the free flow of urine, or prostate enlargement which is also obstructing the free flow of urine. If the prostate is infected with bacteria (chronic bacterial prostatitis), then it becomes a focal point for recurrent infection of the urinary tract (bladder, urethra, etc). These patients may have no signs of prostate enlargement such as those detailed in the questionnaire, but have recurrent infections, usually involving the same micro-organism. This may recur every few months or more frequently, one infection starting almost as soon as the previous one has cleared up. This requires an accurate diagnosis and means consulting a health professional who can do cultures as well as examine the prostate as to its status.

One agent which may be involved in prostatitis is trichomonas vaginalis. This is a protozoa and is spread by sexual transmission from an infected person. Its ability to thrive in an individual will depend upon such factors as local tissue acidity and hormone presence. When it is in an optimum environment for growth, and is able to replicate then it produces inflammation of the mucosal lining of the tissues. In women this may involve the vagina; and in both sexes it may involve the urethra and/or the bladder, and in males the prostate. Symptoms such as itching, burning and red-yellow discharge are noted and depending upon the area either urethritis or prostatitis (or vaginitis) will be found.

The possibility of infection by trichomonas or a bacteria should be born in mind when symptoms such as these are recurrent. If sexually transmitted then all contacts should be appropriately treated to prevent recurrence.

Treatment
Medical treatment of inflammation/infection of the prostate is to attack the bacterial aspect of the problems. This in itself does little apart from stopping the infection for the short-term. It in no way improves the background reasons which allowed the infection to occur. Thus recurrence is more or less assured, and the prospects are less than good for health in the region. The long-term prospect is that the individual might well

find himself a candidate for surgery to remove the prostate. This is a fairly serious operation and is one which can leave the bladder function impaired. In the main it is an unnecessary operation because reduction in size of the prostate is not difficult to achieve by means of the methods outlined previously. Once reduction in size is achieved it will lead eventually to normalization of the bladder-emptying mechanisms, as well as to the correct acidic balance in the urine, thus reducing the chances of infection and of inflammation. This is the logical approach to recurrent urethritis and cystitis.

Whether treating an episode of urethritis, cystitis, prostatitis or pyelitis, the approach is the same. Initially a high dosage of vitamin C should be taken. It is possible to obtain from any pharmacist litmus paper or a self-test kit for assessing the acidity of the urine. If the urine shows itself to be excessively acid, rather than alkaline, and there has been a diagnosis of stones in the bladder or kidneys, then the vitamin C taken should be in the form of sodium ascorbate which will not further increase the acidity of the urine. In such cases it is also suggested that a dose of 100 milligrams of vitamin B6 be taken daily.

If the urine tests as alkaline, which is abnormal since it should always be acid, then the vitamin C should be taken in the form of ascorbic acid, rather than sodium ascorbate. This will acidify the urine, and if phosphate crystals have been forming, these will then dissolve. Again vitamin B6 should be added to the list of supplements.

Summary
The first priority is to find out whether the urine is acidic or alkaline, and then to start taking the appropriate form of vitamin C.

1. Test urine: if *acid* and there is infection, take sodium ascorbate (dosage given below). If *alkaline*, take ascorbic acid (dosage given below). In either case take additional Vitamin B6 (pyridoxine).

2. Dosage: in the case of infection of the bladder, urethra or kidneys it is necessary to achieve what is termed 'saturation' of the tissues with vitamin C. This is achieved by increasing the dose from 3 grams of the appropriate form of vitamin C as determined by the acid/alkaline testing spread throughout the day by 1 gram per day until the bowels react by the beginnings of diarrhoea. When this occurs bowel tolerance has been reached, and the dosage will have gone just beyond saturation requirements. In other words by increasing the dosage daily in this way, the body is tested for its current requirement limit. Each individual differs in the amounts of vitamin C (and all other nutrients) required. We also need different amounts under varying circumstances; infection and stress are two factors which result in a greater requirement of vitamin C than usual. So one of the easiest ways of asking the body how much vitamin C it requires at any time is to follow the pattern described above, until the body itself indicates it has sufficient (the diarrhoea being the signal). The diarrhoea should cease

as soon as the levels of vitamin C being taken are dropped a little. Thus the amount taken on the day previous to the onset of diarrhoea should be resumed and the bowels will normally settle. This level of intake should be maintained until the infection has passed. However it is most important not to suddenly reduce the intake once the symptoms have cleared because a rebound of the infection could occur. The dosage should be restored to normal (1 to 3 grams per day, if prostrate enlargement has been a problem) by reducing the intake by 1 gram per day until this target is reached.

Such a programme of vitamin C supplements is the primary defence measure recommended against infection of the urinary tract. However alongside this should go the taking of zinc and essential fatty acids, as described in the previous chapter. No increase in intake of these is necessary since levels are already adequate for infection, as well as for BPH, as described. (Pollen may be used as a source of EFA's.)

In some cases where it is impossible to pass water it is necessary for catheterization to be performed to relieve the urine build up. This, of course, requires expert nursing attention and is not a self-help measure. Such measures as hot hip baths or hot towels over the pelvic area can also assist in relief of such a pressure build-up, but should this not be rapidly effective, expert advice should be sought from a doctor. Once the build up of urine has been cleared in this way, implementation of the advice given in this and previous chapters, will be found to achieve remarkably rapid improvement. Full recovery of bladder function, as evidenced by the absence of the various symptoms already described, takes months rather than weeks and requires an ongoing commitment through dietary care, even when the symptoms are once again more or less normal.

10.

The Key to Prostate Health

There are different elements relating to diet and its effect on the prostate. Firstly there is what may be termed a detoxification diet. This involves a period, or repeated periods, in which the foods selected should have a cleansing, detoxifying effect on the body as a whole. This could include the use of therapeutic fasting, short periods abstinence from food as such, during which fruit only, juices only, or water only were consumed.

The second aspect of the diet, as it relates to prostate problems, is the use of long-term dietary strategies to provide, in food form, the essential nutrients so important for health in general, and prostate health in particular. Such a diet would need to take account of the importance of a reduction in the cholesterol level of the bloodstream. It would also need to focus on bowel health, so would, of necessity, be a diet high in fibre content. Since this is the type of diet which also protects against diabetes, heart disease and cancer, it can be seen to be a highly desirable dietary pattern.

The third aspect of the diet which has to be considered, is the highlighting of those foods and substances which are undesirable and indeed downright dangerous as far as prostate problems are concerned.

By taking into account these different aspects of diet, a plan of action can be produced which largely eliminates from the diet any positively undesirable substances, as well as incorporating into everyday eating those foods which are rich in the nutrients necessary for prostate health. Into such a pattern it is then possible to build periods of elimination or detoxification which can be introduced weekly, monthly or at whatever interval is preferred, and can last for one to two days or more, depending upon the needs and general health of the individual.

Detoxification

Note: if the person considering such a course of action is very frail or underweight, then advice should be sought prior to commencing from a qualified naturopathic practitioner (address of professional association given below).

Any animal lover will know that when an animal becomes ill its first priority seems to be to rest and to stop all food intake. This is nature's way of allowing the self-healing mechanisms of the body to act unhindered by the requirements of the digestive process, which uses up so much energy and effort.

Fasting creates a period of physiological rest, during which self-healing and repairing mechanisms (called the homoeostatic mechanism) can begin to normalize and restore injured or diseased parts of the body. It is self-evident that when we injure ourselves, the body repairs that damage, all other things being equal. Similarly in ill-health it is the self-repairing effort of the body which restores normality. Treatment is designed to aid that effort by provision of a desirable environment and essential nutrients, whilst at the same time removing any obstacles to recovery. All other treatment is purely palliative, i.e. designed to make the patient more comfortable while recovering. The body heals itself and we must therefore assist in this endeavour by removing any hindrances while hopefully not adding to its burdens, as so many forms of drug treatment unfortunately do.

This is why certain undesirable foods and substances need to be removed from the diet in particular illnesses. In prostate problems this calls for abstinence from alcohol, coffee, refined carbohydrates, saturated fats and all chemicalized foods. It also calls for a series of short fasts or detoxification periods, which can be carried out for one day per week, or for two or three days every month, as preferred. These can be semi-fasts or total fasts, and the choice must to a large extent depend upon the general health of the individual, as well as their circumstances. Someone who is alone and looking after themselves, should choose a semi-fast. If there is someone on hand to cope with odd errands and general help, then a total fast can be chosen, since bed-rest, although not usual, may be needed.

Fasting is the most natural and the oldest of all healing methods 'and has profoundly beneficial effects on the body and its self-healing efforts. However it must be stressed that longer fasts, or fasts by individuals who are in a very frail condition, should only be undertaken when a degree of supervision is available, and advice has been taken from an expert in this field. Also anyone taking drugs should seek advice as to whether a fast is desirable or not.

In semi-fasting, the spring water-only rule of complete fasting is relaxed a little to allow the use of natural unsweetened fruits and juices. When prostate problems arise a semi-fast should be adopted for not less than 24 hours and not more than three days. If a 24-hour period is selected then this should be repeated weekly. It is desirable that during this period a good deal of rest is taken, although bed-rest should only be needed rarely. Normally a person on a semi-fast can walk around and potter although it is best if no serious work is undertaken and that the person does not drive during this time. There is no limit to the amount of juices which can be consumed, although it should not be less than 3 pints a day.

For anyone who is working the ideal time for a semi-fast is at the weekend. Start on Friday night with a light fruit-only meal, then over the next day or two consume only juices such as apple, grape or diluted citrus (50/50 with water) together with plenty of bottled water. If this proves too difficult to follow, try a mono-diet of grapes only as a compromise. After 24 to 48 hours of this the fast or mono-diet should be broken by the eating of a little stewed apple and natural yoghurt (low fat) or a banana. The following meal should be a salad or all fruit meal, then the normal diet can resume.

Anyone who has previously been following a typical modern diet full of refined and undesirable foods will probably note on the first day or so of a fast, some unpleasant symptoms, such as furred tongue, slight nausea, and a headache. This is evidence of the detoxification process getting under way, with the liver attempting to cleanse the body of the wastes being stirred up by the fasting process. Urine will become very dark or cloudy, further evidence of this process. The bowels may not work for a day or so, but this should be of no concern on a short fast as normality will be restored by the body's own efforts. If a longer fast is undertaken and this lack of bowel movement occurs, then an enema is suggested, once daily.

It is not desirable for a water-only fast to be undertaken by anyone inexperienced in these measures, and so guidelines are not given here. A naturopathic practitioner should be consulted for guidance on this.

A semi-fast, repeated weekly or every few weeks, will have a marked effect on general health. Skin will clear and appear more elastic, energy will improve, sleep will be deeper, eyesight and all other senses will be keener, and a multitude of minor symptoms will disappear. All this takes time, however, and is not to be anticipated after one or two fast periods only.

There are no dangers from a semi-fast unless cancer or a diabetic state exists, in which case advice needs to be taken first from a qualified practitioner. (Contact BNOA, 6 Netherhall Gardens, London NW3, for the name of your nearest naturopathic practitioner.)

General Dietary Strategy

In order to produce maximum results for the prostate, a general dietary strategy needs to improve bowel health, reduce cholesterol levels in the blood, and ensure provision of ample zinc, essential fatty acids and other nutrients through daily food intake.

Bowel function should be regular and unstrained. This calls for a high fibre content in the diet. Fibre comes in various guises. There is the obvious roughage of the cereal variety, found in bran and in the outer casing of unrefined grains, such as brown rice, etc. There are also many gentler and more important sources of fibre. These include the gums and mucilages found in fruits, nuts and seeds and in most vegetables, and in all the bean family. These are more effective in removing cholesterol from the blood than the grain-derived fibres (brans, etc), thus high fibre intake of the gum/mucilage variety not only achieves the regular movement of the bowels, but also has a profound anti-cholesterol effect.

Cholesterol is a naturally occurring substance

which the body makes for itself in abundance. This is important to understand, for far from being an enemy of the body, no single cell of the body can function without cholesterol. It is only when excessive amounts, of the wrong type, of cholesterol are found in the body that alarm bells are sounded. This is not always a simple matter of high levels in the body resulting from a high cholesterol level in the diet. In fact it is known that the cholesterol we eat, in eggs for example, plays but a minimal part in the level found in the body. Rather it is the result of the type of fat we eat and of the amount of sugar consumed. When a high level of saturated fat and sugars are part of the diet, cholesterol levels go up.

Again it is a little more complex than it seems because there are different types of cholesterol transporters in the blood, called high density and low density, and very low density, lipoproteins. In simple terms the more harmful types of cholesterol are now known to increase in the bloodstream, and to do harm from there, when the diet is rich in saturated fat and especially when saturated fat and sugar (whatever the colour of the sugar) are a major element of the diet. Other elements in the diet compound this problem, such as a high coffee intake and alcohol. Fibre is an effective way of tackling this problem, and a diet which is low in sugar, low in saturated fat, and high in fibre is an anti-cholesterol diet. This means that it is an anti-prostate cancer diet too.

The major elements required to achieve such a health-inducing diet are whole grains, fresh fruits, nuts and seeds, vegetables, and all the pulses. These must form a major part of the everyday eating pattern of the prostate sufferer, or of anyone who wants to avoid such problems. Foods which contain no fibre are the dairy products and meat and fish. These are not therefore of any use in a fibre-enhancing programme, although some of them are of extreme importance if adequate protein is to be eaten.

Obviously a choice exists as to whether or not a vegetarian diet is followed. Such a dietary pattern has definite advantages for health, providing it is well structured. There is always the danger on a vegetarian diet that inadequate protein intake will occur, but this can be prevented by taking care as to the combination of such elements as grains and pulses (beans) so that all the amino acids necessary for the body to construct its own first-class protein are provided. A vegetarian diet usually allows for an immediate high fibre intake (unless white flour and white sugar products are being inadvisedly eaten), as well as a reduction in the chances of eating excess saturated fat, which is so much part of a diet containing lots of dairy foods and meat.

If a meat-eating diet is selected, then a reduction in saturated fats has to be considered carefully. Selecting fish and poultry (apart from the skin of chicken) and using only low fat dairy products, goes some way to achieving this. Game is a further choice which lowers the risk of saturated fat being eaten – game, such as rabbit, hare or venison contains an average of only 4 per cent of the body weight as fat. Beef often achieves 30 per cent of body weight as fat. The type of fat is also very different in that the fat from cows, pigs and sheep is mainly saturated, whereas the minimal amount of fat in game is largely unsaturated. Also do not be misled into thinking that trimming visible fat from meat will achieve the desired reduction, for much fat in pig, sheep or cow meat is not visible.

Fish is a useful source of desirable fats, especially when cold water fish, such as the herring, is eaten. The essential fatty acids, so necessary to health generally and to the prostate in particular, can be found in many vegetable foods, including seeds such as pumpkin and sunflower, which are also rich in zinc. The green element in vegetables, chlorophyll, is a rich source of vitamins such as A, E and K, as well as essential fatty acids, and so plenty of green vegetables in the diet will add to the balance of these nutrients. Naturally green vegetables also contain (when fresh) a great deal of vitamin C, as well as fibre.

We can see from this appraisal that the type of diet we should aim for should be rich in green vegetables and protein, whether of animal (low saturated fat type) or vegetarian (pulse and grain combinations). It should also incorporate seeds and nuts, which contain other vital elements, and be sparing in dairy produce and the undesirable meats mentioned.

A basic pattern of diet could be as follows:

- *Breakfast*
  Fresh fruit plus a seed and nut mixture (e.g.

sunflower, sesame, pumpkin, linseed together with almonds, walnuts, hazelnuts, etc). These can be ground, crushed or eaten whole as preferred. If chewing is a problem the mixture of seeds, nuts and fruit can be placed into a food processor and reduced to a pulp for easy eating. A seed and nut mixture can also be incorporated with oatflakes and moistened with natural low fat yoghurt or fruit juice.

It provides essential fatty acids and zinc, as well as plenty of protein and fibre.

If still hungry then wholemeal toast and a no-sugar jam with a cup of herbal tea may be eaten.

- *Mid-morning snack* (if required)
Eat fresh fruit or seeds and nuts (also fresh, for beware of such foods if there is any rancidity — nuts are best cracked personally rather than purchasing them ready shelled) and/or drink herbal tea, such as Rooibos, camomile, parsley or lemon verbena.
- *Lunch*
A large mixed salad, incorporating as wide a variety of different vegetables as possible. Green leafy vegetables as well as root vegetables (grated finely) can be made into a mixture which provides different tastes, textures and colours, to tempt even the most jaded of appetites. Raw mushrooms, avocado, and other unusual ingredients can add to this. Together with the vegetables have a mixture of nuts and seeds and cottage or other low fat cheese, as well as a brown rice savoury or a baked potato. If a potato is not eaten, then

wholemeal bread can be added. No butter or margarine should be used, but rather a little olive oil on the potato.

Dress the salad with an olive oil and lemon juice mixture, or with natural low fat yoghurt.

Fresh fruit for dessert.

- *Mid-afternoon snack* (if required)
  As for the mid-morning snack.
- *Evening meal*
  A cooked protein meal based on either fish, poultry or game, together with a variety of seasonal cooked and raw vegetables. The American habit of always having a side salad is to be recommended.

If a vegetarian choice is made for protein, then any of a wide variety of dishes, suitably described in many cook books, can be used. This could include grains (rice, wheat, millet, etc) and pulses (chickpeas, butterbeans, haricot beans, soya beans, lentils, etc). Also of course there are egg dishes and cheese dishes, although cooked cheese is not recommended. (It is, of course, quite in order to reverse the main meal pattern and to have the cooked meal midday and the salad in the evening, if this is preferred or more convenient.)

Fresh fruit or yoghurt for dessert.

Foods to Avoid

Alcohol should be taken very sparingly, if at all. No more than one and a half wineglasses of dry white wine daily is permitted to anyone in good health, if they are hoping to maintain that happy state. If there are prostate problems in evidence, then no alcohol at all should be consumed.

Coffee, in very small amounts only, is permitted for anyone with prostate problems. This means no more than one cup of filtered coffee daily. Boiled coffee increases cholesterol levels and instant coffee does not bear thinking about.

All sugar should be avoided and certainly not consumed as an additive to food, or in the form of sweets, chocolates, pastries, etc.

Saturated fats should also be considered undesirable. These are found in all animal fats and in most margarine, as well as in all foods which have been fried.

All foods which have been contaminated by pesticides, or in which artifical colouring, flavouring or other additives have been used should be avoided. Another reason for avoiding animal meats from most farm sources is the inclusion in their diets of hormones which enhance their growth. Some residues of these pass into the body of the person eating the meat, and since these are largely of female hormone origin, they would increase the dangers of prostate enlargement by suppressing testosterone activity.

By following the type of diet outlined here, together with occasional semi-fasts, and ensuring adequate supplies of nutrients as described in previous chapters, the health of the prostate will be restored to as near normal as is possible. In many cases this will be completely normal.

It might appear that there are many elements which all require attention, but concentration on the basic diet, together with the important nutrient supplements discussed (available from most health food stores) will rapidly produce improvement. The use of the hydrotherapy and prostate massage methods are not essential but offer a degree of extra assistance which can ease the process of recovery which the diet will ensure.

These methods are not designed for use in prostate cancer, although there is little doubt that the basic dietary and supplement approach will improve such a condition, to the extent that this is possible. Surgery in such a case might be advisable, since if there has been no spread of the cancer, excision of the gland can contain the problem. Prevention is by far the better policy, and the use of the dietary methods presented will give this a strong chance.

Prostate problems are *not* inevitable and are mainly curable by self-help measures. This claim is based on countless cases of recovery from benign prostatic hypertrophy and its complications of cystitis, urethritis and prostatitis.

Index